52 Vitamin Packed Lung Cancer Juice Recipes:

Powerful Ingredient Combinations That Will Help Your Body Destroy Cancer Cells

By

Joe Correa CSN

COPYRIGHT

This publication is designed to provide accurate and authoritative information in regard to the subject matter covered. It is sold with the understanding that neither the author nor the publisher is engaged in rendering medical advice. If medical advice or assistance is needed, consult with a doctor. This book is considered a guide and should not be used in any way detrimental to your health. Consult with a physician before starting this nutritional plan to make sure it's right for you.

ACKNOWLEDGEMENTS

This book is dedicated to my friends and family that have had mild or serious illnesses so that you may find a solution and make the necessary changes in your life.

52 Vitamin Packed Lung Cancer Juice Recipes:

Powerful Ingredient Combinations That Will Help Your Body Destroy Cancer Cells

By

Joe Correa CSN

CONTENTS

ABOUT THE AUTHOR

After years of Research, I honestly believe in the positive effects that proper nutrition can have over the body and mind. My knowledge and experience has helped me live healthier throughout the years and which I have shared with family and friends. The more you know about eating and drinking healthier, the sooner you will want to change your life and eating habits.

Nutrition is a key part in the process of being healthy and living longer so get started today. The first step is the most important and the most significant.

INTRODUCTION

52 Vitamin Packed Lung Cancer Juice Recipes: Powerful Ingredient Combinations That Will Help Your Body Destroy Cancer Cells

By Joe Correa CSN

Food has a big impact on our body and our health. Almost all diseases are directly related to the foods we eat which is why it's crucial to choose carefully what we put at the table. It has the power to heal our bodies from within, which is especially important for people who have lung cancer or any type of cancer. Sometimes, we consume unnatural quantities of pharmaceuticals that may or may not be effective which can ultimately weaken our immune system and our entire body.

In this book, I will share with you some valuable juice recipes that will give your body the nutrients it needs in order to function properly and fight off all types of diseases. Implementing these recipes into your everyday life will have a powerful effect on your overall health. I honestly believe we have no choice but to forge our own path to wellness through adequate food choices. This primarily refers to fresh fruits and vegetables which are the key to good health. The more we are able to return to eating as nature intended, the better our chances will be of living a cancer-free life.

When we talk about lung cancer, your best options are colorful fruits and vegetables. These foods are full of antioxidants, including vitamins A and C which are proven to help fight off this type of cancer. Fruits like berries and vegetables like tomatoes, winter squash, and bell peppers are particularly good and your juices should be based on them. These foods, when combined correctly, can be very delicious.

Having this in mind, I have created a wonderful collection of lung cancer preventing juice recipes that are tasty and effective. Have fun trying them all!

52 VITAMIN PACKED LUNG CANCER JUICE RECIPES: POWERFUL INGREDIENT COMBINATIONS THAT WILL HELP YOUR BODY DESTROY CANCER CELLS

1.   **Spinach Broccoli Juice**

Ingredients:

1 cup of fresh spinach, torn

1 cup of broccoli, chopped

1 small Granny Smith's apple, cored

1 cup of green grapes

1 tbsp fresh mint, finely chopped

Preparation:

Using a large colander, rinse the spinach and broccoli under cold running water. Slightly drain and torn the spinach in small pieces. Trim off the outer leaves of the broccoli and cut into small pieces. Fill the measuring cups and set aside.

Wash the apple and cut lengthwise in half. Remove the core and cut into bite-sized pieces. Set aside.

Wash the grapes and remove the stem. Set aside.

Now, combine spinach, broccoli, apple, and grapes in a juicer and process until well juiced. Transfer to a serving glass and sprinkle with some fresh mint.

Refrigerate for 10 minutes before serving.

Nutrition information per serving: Kcal: 176, Protein: 9.8g, Carbs: 49.5g, Fats: 1.7g

2. Blueberry Beet Juice

Ingredients:

1 cup of blueberries

1 whole lime, peeled

1 large banana, sliced

1 cup of Romaine lettuce, shredded

1 whole cucumber, sliced

Preparation:

Rinse the blueberries using a small colander. Slightly drain and fill the measuring cup. Set aside.

Peel the lime and cut lengthwise in half. Set aside.

Peel the banana and cut into thin slices. Set aside.

Rinse the lettuce thoroughly under cold running water. Shred it and fill the measuring cup. Set aside.

Wash the cucumber and cut into thin slices. Set aside.

Now, combine blueberries, lime, banana, lettuce, and cucumber in a juicer and process until juiced. Transfer to a serving glass and add some crushed ice.

Serve immediately.

Nutrition information per serving: Kcal: 176, Protein: 9.8g, Carbs: 49.5g, Fats: 1.7g

3.   Avocado Beet Juice

Ingredients:

1 cup of avocado, chopped

1 cup of beets, trimmed

1 large carrot, sliced

1 small ginger knob

¼ tsp turmeric, ground

2 oz water

Preparation:

Peel the avocado and cut lengthwise in half. Remove the pit and cut into bite-sized pieces. Fill the measuring cup and reserve the rest in the refrigerator.

Trim off the green parts of the beets. Slightly peel and cut into thin slices. Fill the measuring cup and refrigerate the rest.

Wash and peel the carrot. Cut into bite-sized pieces and set aside.

Peel the ginger knob and cut into small pieces. Set aside.

Now, combine avocado, beets, carrot, and ginger in a juicer. Process until well juiced and transfer to a serving glass. Stir in the turmeric and water and refrigerate for 15 minutes before serving.

Enjoy!

Nutrition information per serving: Kcal: 265, Protein: 5.9g, Carbs: 33.4g, Fats: 21.8g

4. Pomegranate Cantaloupe Juice

Ingredients:

1 cup of pomegranate seeds

1 large wedge of cantaloupe

1 small green apple, cored

1 small ginger knob, sliced

1 oz of water

Preparation:

Cut the top of the pomegranate fruit using a sharp paring knife. Slice down to each of the white membranes inside of the fruit. Pop the seeds into a measuring cup and set aside.

Cut the cantaloupe in half. Scrape out the seeds and cut one one large wedge. Peel and chop into small pieces. Wrap the rest in a plastic foil and refrigerate for later.

Wash the apple and cut lengthwise in half. Remove the core and cut into bite-sized pieces. Set aside.

Peel the ginger and cut into small pieces. Set aside.

Now, combine pomegranate, cantaloupe, apple, and ginger in a juicer. Process until well juiced and transfer to a serving glass. Add some water to adjust the bitterness, if needed.

Refrigerate for 10-15 minutes before serving.

Nutrition information per serving: Kcal: 162, Protein: 3.1g, Carbs: 45.3g, Fats: 1.5g

5.   Grapefruit Apricot Juice

Ingredients:

2 whole grapefruits

1 cup of collard greens, chopped

2 whole apricots, pitted

¼ tsp of turmeric, ground

Preparation:

Peel the grapefruits and divide into wedges. Cut each wedge in half and set aside.

Wash the collard greens thoroughly under cold running water. Drain and chop into small pieces. Set aside.

Wash the apricots and cut lengthwise in half. Remove the pit and cut into bite-sized pieces. Set aside.

Now, combine grapefruit, collard greens, and apricots in a juicer and process until juiced. Transfer to a serving glass and stir in the turmeric.

Refrigerate for 10 minutes before serving.

Enjoy!

Nutrition information per serving: Kcal: 208, Protein: 5.8g, Carbs: 62.1g, Fats: 1.2g

6.   Honeydew Melon Cucumber Juice

Ingredients:

1 large wedge of honeydew melon

1 cup of cucumber, sliced

1 cup of whole cranberries

2 large strawberries

1 oz coconut water

Preparation:

Cut melon lengthwise in half. Scoop out the seeds and then wash the melon. Cut one wedge and peel it. Cut into bite-sized pieces and set aside.

Wash the cucumber and cut into thin slices. Fill the measuring cup and reserve the rest for later. Set aside.

Using a small colander, rinse well the cranberries. Drain and set aside.

Wash the strawberries and remove the stems. Chop into small pieces and set aside.

Now, combine melon, cucumber, cranberries, and strawberries in a juicer. Process until well juiced. Transfer to a serving glass and add few ice cubes.

Serve immediately.

Nutrition information per serving: Kcal: 96, Protein: 1.8g, Carbs: 31.4g, Fats: 0.6g

7.   Cauliflower Artichoke Juice

Ingredients:

1 cup of cauliflower, chopped

1 medium artichoke, chopped

1 whole lemon, peeled and halved

1 small zucchini, thinly sliced

1 small ginger knob, chopped

¼ tsp salt

Preparation:

Trim off the outer layer of the cauliflower. Cut into bite-sized pieces and wash it. Fill the measuring cup and sprinkle with some salt. Set aside.

Trim off the outer layers of the artichoke using a sharp paring knife. Cut into bite-sized pieces and set aside.

Peel the lemon and cut lengthwise in half. Set aside.

Wash the zucchini and thinly slice it. Set aside.

Peel the ginger knob and chop into small pieces. Set aside.

Now, combine cauliflower, artichoke, lemon, zucchini, and ginger in a juicer. Process until well juiced.

Transfer to a serving glass and refrigerate for 15 minutes before serving.

Enjoy!

Nutrition information per serving: Kcal: 82, Protein: 8.4g, Carbs: 28.9g, Fats: 1.1g

8.   Pineapple Banana Juice

Ingredients:

1 cup of pineapple chunks

1 large banana, sliced

1 cup of blackberries

1 whole lime, peeled

1 oz of water

Preparation:

Using a sharp paring knife, cut the top of the pineapple. Gently remove all hard skin and slice it into thin slices. Fill the measuring cup and reserve the rest for later.

Peel the banana and cut into thin slices. Set aside.

Place the blackberries in a small colander and wash under cold running water. Slightly drain and set aside.

Peel the lime and cut lengthwise in half. Set aside.

Now, combine pineapple, banana, blackberries, and lime in a juicer. Process until well juiced. Transfer to a serving glass and add some ice before serving.

Enjoy!

Nutrition information per serving: Kcal: 222, Protein: 4.5g, Carbs: 70.2g, Fats: 1.4g

9.   Bell Pepper Tomato Juice

Ingredients:

1 large red bell pepper, chopped

1 medium whole tomato, chopped

1 cup of watercress, torn

1 rosemary sprig

1 oz of water

Preparation:

Wash the bell pepper and cut lengthwise in half. Remove the seeds and chop into small pieces. Set aside.

Wash the tomato and place in a small bowl. Chop into small pieces and make sure to reserve the tomato juice while cutting. Set aside.

Wash the watercress thoroughly under cold running water. Slightly drain and torn with hands into small pieces. Set aside.

Now, combine bell pepper, tomato, and watercress in a juicer and process until juiced. Transfer to a serving glass and stir in the water and reserved tomato juice. Sprinkle with rosemary and serve immediately.

Enjoy!

Nutrition information per serving: Kcal: 56, Protein: 3.5g, Carbs: 15.1g, Fats: 0.7g

10.   Pumpkin Carrot Juice

Ingredients:

1 cup of pumpkin, cubed

1 large carrot, sliced

1 cup of cucumber, sliced

1 large orange, peeled and wedged

1 small ginger knob, chopped

Preparation:

Cut the top of a pumpkin. Cut lengthwise in half and then scrape out the seeds. Cut one large wedge and peel it. Cut into small cubes and fill the measuring cup. Reserve the rest in the refrigerator.

Wash and peel the carrot. Cut into thin slices and set aside.

Wash the cucumber and cut into thin slices. Fill the measuring cup and reserve the rest for later. Set aside.

Peel the orange and divide into wedges. Cut each wedge in half and set aside.

Peel the ginger knob and cut into small pieces. Set aside.

Now, combine pumpkin, carrot, cucumber, orange, and ginger in a juicer. Process until well juiced. Transfer to a serving glass and add some ice.

Serve immediately.

Nutrition information per serving: Kcal: 130, Protein: 4.1g, Carbs: 39.1g, Fats: 0.6g

11.　　Spinach Radish Juice

Ingredients:

1 cup of fresh spinach, torn

2 large radishes, chopped

1 cup of cucumber, sliced

1 cup of arugula, torn

¼ tsp turmeric, ground

Preparation:

Wash the spinach thoroughly under cold running water. Slightly drain and torn with hands. Set aside.

Wash the radishes and trim off the green parts. Peel and cut into thin slices. Set aside.

Wash the cucumber and cut into thin slices. Set aside.

Wash the arugula and torn with hands. Set aside.

Now, combine spinach, radish, cucumber, and arugula in a juicer and process until juiced. Transfer to a serving glass and stir in the turmeric.

Refrigerate for 15 minutes before serving.

Nutrition information per serving: Kcal: 53, Protein: 9.4g, Carbs: 15.3g, Fats: 1.1g

12.   Apple Plum Juice

Ingredients:

1 medium-sized Red Delicious apple, cored

1 whole plum, cored

1 large banana, peeled and chunked

¼ tsp of cinnamon, ground

2 oz of water

Preparation:

Wash the apple and cut lengthwise in half. Remove the core and cut into bite-sized pieces. Set aside.

Wash the plum and cut in half. Remove the pit and cut into bite-sized pieces. Set aside.

Peel the banana and cut into small chunks. Set aside.

Now, combine apple, plum, and banana in a juicer and process until well juiced. Transfer to a serving glass and stir in the water and cinnamon.

Add few ice cubes before serving and enjoy!

Nutrition information per serving: Kcal: 238, Protein: 2.5g, Carbs: 68.4g, Fats: 1.1g

13. Broccoli Beet Juice

Ingredients:

2 cups of broccoli, chopped

1 cup of beets, trimmed and chopped

1 cup of fresh parsley, torn

1 cup of celery, chopped

¼ tsp of turmeric, ground

¼ tsp ginger, ground

Preparation:

Wash the broccoli and trim off the outer layers. Chop into small pieces and set aside.

Wash and peel the beets. Trim off the green ends and chop into bite-sized pieces. Fill the measuring cup and reserve the rest for later.

Rinse the parsley under cold running water and slightly drain. Torn with hands into small pieces and set aside.

Wash the celery stalks and chop it into bite-sized pieces. Fill the measuring cup and set aside.

Now, combine broccoli, beets, parsley, and celery in a juicer and process until juiced. Transfer to a serving glass and stir in the turmeric and ginger.

Refrigerate for 10 minutes before serving.

Nutrition information per serving: Kcal: 109, Protein: 9.8g, Carbs: 31.8g, Fats: 1.5g

14.   Watermelon Peach Juice

Ingredients:

1 cup of watermelon, cubed

1 large peach, pitted and chopped

1 medium-sized green apple, cored and chopped

1 small banana, chunked

¼ tsp of cinnamon, ground

Preparation:

Cut the watermelon in half. Cut one large wedge and wrap the rest in a plastic foil and refrigerate. Peel the slice and cut into small cubes. Remove the pits and fill the measuring cup. Set aside.

Wash the peach and cut lengthwise in half. Remove the pit and chop into bite-sized pieces. Set aside.

Peel the banana and cut into small chunks. Set aside.

Now, combine watermelon, peach, apple, and banana in a juicer and process until juiced. Transfer to a serving glass and stir in the cinnamon.

Add some ice and serve immediately!

Nutrition information per serving: Kcal: 260, Protein: 4.4g, Carbs: 73.9g, Fats: 1.3g

15.   Yellow Pepper Zucchini Juice

Ingredients:

1 large yellow bell pepper, chopped

1 medium-sized zucchini, sliced

1 cup of fresh basil, chopped

1 large carrot, sliced

¼ tsp of ginger, ground

Preparation:

Wash the bell pepper and cut lengthwise in half. Remove the stem and seeds. Cut into small pieces and set aside.

Wash the zucchini and cut into small chunks. Set aside.

Wash the basil thoroughly under cold running water. Slightly drain and chop into small pieces. Set aside.

Wash and peel the carrot. Cut into thin slices and set aside.

Now, combine pepper, zucchini, basil, and carrot in a juicer and process until juiced. Transfer to a serving glass and stir in the ginger. Add some water if needed.

Refrigerate for 10 minutes before serving.

Nutrition information per serving: Kcal: 94, Protein: 5.6g, Carbs: 25.4g, Fats: 1.3g

16.   Strawberry Spinach Juice

Ingredients:

1 cup of strawberries, chopped

1 cup of spinach, torn

1 whole lemon, peeled

1 whole lime, peeled

1 tbsp honey, raw

2 oz of water

Preparation:

Wash the strawberries and remove the stems. Cut into bite-sized pieces and set aside.

Wash the spinach thoroughly under cold running water. Slightly drain and torn into small pieces. Set aside.

Peel the lemon and lime. Cut each fruit lengthwise in half and set aside.

Now, combine strawberries, spinach, lemon, and lime in a juicer and process until juiced. Transfer to a serving glass and stir in the water and honey.

Garnish with some mint, but it's optional.

Refrigerate for 15 minutes before serving.

Enjoy!

Nutrition information per serving: Kcal: 81, Protein: 5.8g, Carbs: 27.8g, Fats: 1.4g

17.   Asparagus Cauliflower Juice

Ingredients:

1 cup of asparagus, chopped

1 cup of cauliflower, chopped

1 cup of celery, chopped

1 cup of cucumber, sliced

¼ tsp of turmeric, ground

¼ tsp of cayenne pepper, ground

Preparation:

Wash the asparagus under cold running water. Trim off the woody ends and chop into bite-sized pieces. Set aside.

Wash the cauliflower and trim off the outer leaves. Chop into small pieces and fill the measuring cup. Reserve the rest for later.

Wash the celery and chop into bite-sized pieces. Set aside.

Wash the cucumber and cut into thin slices. Fill the measuring cup and reserve the rest in the refrigerator.

Now, combine asparagus, cauliflower, celery, and cucumber in a juicer and process until juiced. Transfer to a serving glass and stir in the turmeric and cayenne pepper.

Serve immediately.

Nutrition information per serving: Kcal: 52, Protein: 6.1g, Carbs: 15.4g, Fats: 0.7g

18.   Cherry Lemon Juice

Ingredients:

1 cup of fresh cherries, pitted

1 whole lemon, peeled

1 medium-sized artichoke, chopped

1 medium-sized apple, cored

¼ tsp of cinnamon, ground

Preparation:

Wash the cherries using a large colander. Cut each in half and remove the pits. Set aside.

Peel the lemon and cut lengthwise in half. Set aside.

Wash the artichoke and trim off the outer, hard leaves. Cut into bite-sized pieces and set aside.

Wash the apple and cut lengthwise in half. Remove the core and cut into bite-sized pieces. Set aside.

Now, combine cherries, lemon, artichoke, and apple in a juicer and process until juiced. Transfer to a serving glass and stir in the cinnamon.

Refrigerate for 10 minutes before serving.

Nutrition information per serving: Kcal: 205, Protein: 7.2g, Carbs: 66.2g, Fats: 0.9g

19.   Mango Blackberry Juice

Ingredients:

1 cup of mango, chunked

1 cup of blackberries

1 large banana, chunked

1 large orange, peeled

¼ tsp of cinnamon, ground

Preparation:

Wash the mango and cut into small chunks. Fill the measuring cup and reserve the rest for later.

Place the blackberries in a colander and wash under cold running water. Slightly drain and set aside.

Peel the banana and cut into small chunks. Set aside.

Peel the orange and divide into wedges. Cut each wedge in half and set aside.

Now, combine mango, blackberries, banana, and orange in a juicer and process until juiced. Transfer to a serving glass and stir in the cinnamon.

Add few ice cubes and serve immediately.

Nutrition information per serving: Kcal: 296, Protein: 6.6g, Carbs: 91.2g, Fats: 2.1g

20.   Avocado Carrot Juice

Ingredients:

1 cup of avocado, chunked

1 large carrot, chopped

1 cup of collard greens, torn

1 cup of Romaine lettuce, shredded

1 whole cucumber, sliced

¼ tsp of ginger, ground

Preparation:

Peel the avocado and cut lengthwise in half. Remove the pit and cut into small chunks. Fill the measuring cup and reserve the rest in the refrigerator.

Wash and peel the carrot. Cut into thin slices and set aside.

Combine collard greens and lettuce in a large colander. Wash thoroughly under cold running water. Drain and shred. Set aside.

Wash the cucumber and cut into thin slices. Fill the measuring cup and reserve the rest for later. Set aside.

Now, combine avocado, carrot, collard greens, lettuce, and cucumber in a juicer and process until juiced. Transfer to a serving glass and stir in the ginger.

Refrigerate for 10 minutes before serving.

Nutrition information per serving: Kcal: 271, Protein: 7.3g, Carbs: 34.1g, Fats: 22.8g

21.   Raspberry Pear Juice

Ingredients:

1 cup of raspberries

1 large pear, cored

1 whole plum, pitted and chopped

1 medium-sized Granny Smith's apple, cored

¼ tsp of cinnamon, ground

1 oz of coconut water

Preparation:

Wash the raspberries using a small colander. Slightly drain and set aside.

Wash the pear and cut lengthwise in half. Remove the core and cut into small pieces. Set aside.

Wash the plum and cut in half. Remove the pit and set aside.

Wash the apple and cut in half. Remove the core and cut into bite-sized pieces. Set aside.

Now, combine raspberries, pear, plum, and apple in a juicer and process until well juiced. Transfer to a serving glass and stir in the cinnamon and coconut water. Add some crushed ice and serve immediately.

Enjoy!

Nutrition information per serving: Kcal: 239, Protein: 3.5g, Carbs: 79.9g, Fats: 1.6g

22.   Guava Mango Juice

Ingredients:

1 whole guava, chopped

1 cup of mango, chunked

1 tbsp of liquid honey

1 whole lime, peeled

1 cup of cucumber, sliced

1 medium-sized Golden Delicious apple, cored

Preparation:

Peel the guava using a sharp paring knife. Cut into bite-sized pieces and set aside.

Wash and peel the mango. Cut into small chunks and set aside.

Peel the lime and cut lengthwise in half. Set aside.

Wash the cucumber and cut into thin slices. fill the measuring cup and reserve the rest in the refrigerator.

Wash the apple and cut lengthwise in half. Remove the core and cut into bite-sized pieces. Set aside.

Now, combine guava, mango, lime, cucumber, and apple in a juicer and process until well juiced. Transfer to a serving glass and stir in the honey. Add some crushed ice and serve immediately.

Nutrition information per serving: Kcal: 211, Protein: 3.7g, Carbs: 61.1g, Fats: 1.5g

23.   Blueberry Spinach Juice

Ingredients:

1 cup of blueberries

1 cup of fresh spinach, chopped

1 whole lime, peeled

1 medium-sized orange

1 oz coconut water

Preparation:

Place the blueberries in a colander and wash under cold running water. Slightly drain and set aside.

Wash the spinach thoroughly and drain. Chop into small pieces and set aside.

Peel the lime and cut lengthwise in half. Set aside.

Peel the orange and divide into wedges. Cut each wedge in half and set aside.

Now, combine blueberries, spinach, lime, and orange in a juicer and process until well juiced. Transfer to a serving glass and stir in the coconut water.

Sprinkle with some fresh mint. However, it's optional.

Enjoy!

Nutrition information per serving: Kcal: 158, Protein: 8.5g, Carbs: 48.1g, Fats: 1.5g

24.   Pepper Broccoli Juice

Ingredients:

1 large green bell pepper, chopped

1 cup of broccoli, chopped

1 cup of Brussels sprouts, halved

1 whole lime, peeled

2 large carrots, sliced

¼ tsp turmeric, ground

Preparation:

Wash the bell pepper and cut lengthwise in half. Remove the stem and seeds. Chop into small pieces and set aside.

Wash the broccoli and Brussels sprouts. Trim off the wilted and outer leaves. Place in a heavy-bottomed pot and add water enough to cover all. Bring it to a boil and then remove from the heat. Drain well and chop into small pieces. Set aside to cool completely.

Peel the lime and cut lengthwise in half. Set aside.

Wash and peel the carrots. Cut into thin slices and set aside.

Now, combine bell pepper, broccoli, Brussels sprouts, lime, and carrots in a juicer and process until juiced. Transfer to a serving glasses and stir in the turmeric. Add some water, if needed.

Sprinkle with some salt, but it's optional.

Nutrition information per serving: Kcal: 122, Protein: 8.5g, Carbs: 39.1g, Fats: 1.2g

25.   Cantaloupe Grapefruit Juice

Ingredients:

1 cup of cantaloupe, cubed

1 whole grapefruit

1 cup of fresh mint, torn

¼ tsp of cinnamon, ground

1 oz coconut water

Preparation:

Cut the cantaloupe in half. Scoop out the seeds and flesh. Cut and peel one large wedge. Chop into chunks and fill the measuring cup. Reserve the rest of the cantaloupe in a refrigerator.

Peel the grapefruit and divide into wedges. Cut each wedge in half and set aside.

Wash the mint thoroughly and torn with hands into small pieces. Set aside.

Now, combine cantaloupe, grapefruit, and mint in a juicer. Process until well juiced.

Transfer to a serving glass and stir in the cinnamon and coconut water. Add some ice and serve immediately.

Nutrition information per serving: Kcal: 144, Protein: 4.2g, Carbs: 42.6g, Fats: 0.9g

26.   Pomegranate Apple Juice

Ingredients:

1 cup of pomegranate seeds

1 medium-sized Granny Smith's apple, cored

1 large banana, chunked

1 tbsp of liquid honey

1 oz of water

Preparation:

Cut the top of the pomegranate fruit using a sharp paring knife. Slice down to each of the white membranes inside of the fruit. Pop the seeds into a measuring cup and set aside.

Wash the apple and cut lengthwise in half. Remove the core and cut into bite-sized pieces. Set aside.

Peel the banana and cut into small chunks. Set aside.

Now, combine pomegranate, apple, and banana in a juicer and process until juiced. Transfer to a serving glass and stir in the honey and water.

Serve cold.

Nutrition information per serving: Kcal: 243, Protein: 3.6g, Carbs: 70.1g, Fats: 1.8g

27. Zucchini Basil Juice

Ingredients:

1 medium-sized zucchini, chopped

1 cup of fresh basil, torn

1 cup of cucumber, sliced

1 cup of red leaf lettuce, torn

1 cup of avocado, cut into bite-sized pieces

Preparation:

Peel the zucchini and chop into small pieces. Set aside.

Combine basil and lettuce in a large colander and rinse under cold running water. Drain and torn with hands into small pieces. Set aside.

Peel the avocado and cut lengthwise in half. Remove the pit and cut into bite-sized pieces. Fill the measuring cup and reserve the rest in the refrigerator.

Wash the cucumber and cut into thin slices. Fill the measuring cup and refrigerate for later.

Now, combine zucchini, basil, lettuce, avocado, and cucumber in a juicer. Process until well juiced. Transfer to a serving glass and add some ice.

Serve immediately.

Nutrition information per serving: Kcal: 234, Protein: 6.7g, Carbs: 21.7g, Fats: 22.3g

28.   Banana Peach Juice

Ingredients:

1 cup of banana, sliced

1 large peach, pitted and chopped

1 small green apple, cored and chopped

¼ tsp of cinnamon, ground

1 oz of coconut water

1 tbsp of mint, finely chopped

Preparation:

Peel the bananas and cut into thin slices. Fill the measuring cup and reserve the rest in the refrigerator.

Wash the peach and cut lengthwise in half. Remove the pit and cut into bite-sized pieces. Set side.

Wash the apple and cut in half. Remove the core and chop into small pieces. Set aside.

Now, combine bananas, peach, and apple in a juicer and process until well juiced. Transfer to a serving glass and stir in the cinnamon and coconut water. Add some crushed ice and sprinkle with finely chopped mint for some extra taste.

Enjoy!

Nutrition information per serving: Kcal: 362, Protein: 5.5g, Carbs: 104g, Fats: 1.7g

29.   Swiss Chard-Tomato Juice

Ingredients:

1 cup of cherry tomatoes, halved

1 cup of Swiss chard, torn

1 cup of basil, torn

1 cup of beets, trimmed

¼ tsp of balsamic vinegar

¼ tsp of salt

1 oz of water

Preparation:

Wash the cherry tomatoes and remove the green stems. Cut in half and fill the measuring cup. Reserve the rest in the refrigerator for some other juice.

Combine Swiss chard and basil in a large colander and rinse thoroughly under cold running water. Drain and torn with hands into small pieces. Set aside.

Wash the beets and trim off the green parts. Cut into thin slices and fill the measuring cup. Reserve the rest for later.

Now, combine cherry tomatoes, Swiss chard, basil, and beets in a juicer and process until juiced. Transfer to a serving glass and stir in the vinegar, salt, and water.

Serve immediately.

Nutrition information per serving: Kcal: 72, Protein: 5.1g, Carbs: 21.6g, Fats: 0.7g

30.   Pear Apricot Juice

Ingredients:

1 large pear, chopped

3 whole apricots, pitted

1 cup of pomegranate seeds

1 medium-sized orange, wedged

¼ tsp of cinnamon, ground

Preparation:

Wash the pear and cut lengthwise in half. Cut into bite-sized pieces and set aside.

Wash the apricots and cut each in half. Remove the pit and cut into small pieces. Set aside.

Cut the top of the pomegranate fruit using a sharp paring knife. Slice down to each of the white membranes inside of the fruit. Pop the seeds into a measuring cup and set aside.

Peel the orange and divide into wedges. Cut each wedge in half and set aside.

Now, combine pear, apricots, pomegranate seeds, and orange in a juicer. Process until well juiced. Transfer to a serving glass and stir in the cinnamon.

Refrigerate for 10 minutes before serving.

Nutrition information per serving: Kcal: 253, Protein: 4.9g, Carbs: 78.3g, Fats: 1.9g

31. Kale Zucchini Juice

Ingredients:

1 cup of fresh kale, chopped

1 medium-sized zucchini, chopped

1 whole lemon, peeled

1 whole lime, peeled

1 cup of fresh mint, torn

Preparation:

Rinse the kale thoroughly under cold running water. Drain and chop into small pieces. Set aside.

Wash the zucchini and cut into small pieces. Set aside.

Peel the lemon and lime. Cut lengthwise in half and set aside.

Wash the mint and chop into small pieces. Set aside.

Now, combine kale, zucchini, lemon, lime, and mint in a juicer. Process until well juiced. Transfer to a serving glass and add some crushed ice.

Serve immediately.

Nutrition information per serving: Kcal: 79, Protein: 7g, Carbs: 24.7g, Fats: 1.7g

32.   Kiwi Apricot Juice

Ingredients:

2 whole kiwis, peeled and halved

3 whole apricots, chopped

1 large green apple, cored

1 large banana, chunked

Preparation:

Peel the kiwi and cut lengthwise in half. Set aside.

Wash the apricots and cut in half. Remove the pits and cut into small pieces. Set aside.

Wash the apple and cut lengthwise in half. Remove the core and cut into bite-sized pieces. Set aside.

Peel the banana and cut into small chunks. Set aside.

Now, combine kiwi, apricots, apple, and banana in a juicer and process until juiced. Transfer to a serving glass and add some ice.

Serve immediately.

Nutrition information per serving: Kcal: 313, Protein: 5.4g, Carbs: 91g, Fats: 1.9g

33.   Mango Mint Juice

Ingredients:

1 cup of mango, chunked

1 cup of fresh mint, torn

1 small Red Delicious apple, cored

1 medium-sized peach, pitted

Preparation:

Peel the mango and cut into small chunks. Fill the measuring cup and reserve the rest in the refrigerator.

Wash the mint thoroughly under cold running water and torn with hands. Set aside. You can soak mint in hot water for 2 minutes, but it's optional.

Wash the apple and cut lengthwise in half. Remove the core and cut into bite-sized pieces. Set aside.

Wash the peach and cut in half. Remove the pit and cut into small pieces. Set aside.

Now, combine mango, mint, apple, and peach in a juicer and process until well juiced. Transfer to a serving glass and add few ice cubes.

Serve immediately.

Nutrition information per serving: Kcal: 227, Protein: 4.1g, Carbs: 64.9g, Fats: 1.6g

34.   Orange Fennel Juice

Ingredients:

1 medium-sized orange, peeled

1 medium-sized pear, chopped

1 cup of fennel, chopped

1 whole lemon, peeled

¼ tsp of cinnamon, ground

1 oz of coconut water

Preparation:

Peel the orange and divide into wedges. Cut each wedge in half and set aside.

Wash the pear and cut in half. Remove the core and cut into small pieces. Set aside.

Trim off the outer wilted layers of the fennel. Roughly chop it and fill the measuring cup. Reserve the rest for later.

Peel the lemon and cut lengthwise in half. Set aside.

Now, combine orange, pear, fennel, and lemon in a juicer and process until well juiced. Transfer to a serving glass and stir in the cinnamon and coconut water.

Refrigerate for 15 minutes before serving.

Enjoy!

Nutrition information per serving: Kcal: 156, Protein: 3.6g, Carbs: 54.2g, Fats: 0.7g

35.   Beet Raspberry Juice

Ingredients:

1 cup of beets, sliced

1 cup of raspberries

1 whole lemon, peeled

1 medium-sized pear, chopped

1 oz of water

Preparation:

Wash the beets and trim off the green parts. Cut into thin slices and fill the measuring cup. Reserve the rest for later.

Rinse well the raspberries using a small colander. Drain and set aside.

Peel the lemon and cut lengthwise in half. Set aside.

Wash the pear and cut in half. Remove the core and cut into bite-sized pieces. Set aside.

Now, combine beets, raspberries, lemon, and pear in a juicer and process until juiced. Transfer to a serving glass and stir in the water.

Refrigerate for 10 minutes before serving.

Nutrition information per serving: Kcal: 165, Protein: 4.9g, Carbs: 60.2g, Fats: 1.4g

36.   Sweet Potato Celery Juice

Ingredients:

1 cup of sweet potatoes, cubed

1 cup of celery, chopped

1 medium-sized apple, cored

1 medium-sized orange, peeled

1 tbsp of fresh mint, torn

Preparation:

Peel the sweet potato and cut into small cubes. Fill the measuring cup and reserve the rest for later. Set aside.

Wash the celery and cut into bite-sized pieces. Set aside.

Wash the apple and cut lengthwise in half. Remove the core and cut into bite-sized pieces. Set aside.

Peel the orange and divide into wedges. Cut each wedge in half and set aside.

Now, combine sweet potatoes, celery, apple, and orange in a juicer. Process until well juiced. Transfer to a serving glass and sprinkle with mint.

Add some crushed ice and serve immediately.

Nutrition information per serving: Kcal: 236, Protein: 4.7g, Carbs: 67.8g, Fats: 0.7g

37.   Tomato Spinach Juice

Ingredients:

1 medium whole tomato, chopped

1 cup of fresh spinach, torn

1 medium-sized carrot, sliced

1 cup of celery, chopped

¼ tsp of salt

¼ tsp of balsamic vinegar

Preparation:

Wash the tomato and place in a small bowl. Cut into bite-sized pieces. Make sure to reserve the tomato juice while cutting. Set aside.

Wash the spinach thoroughly under cold running water. Torn into small pieces and set aside.

Wash and peel the carrot. Cut into thin slices and set aside.

Wash the celery and chop into small pieces. Set aside.

Now, combine tomato, spinach, carrot, and celery in a juicer and process until juiced. Transfer to a serving glass and stir in the salt, vinegar, and reserved tomato juice.

Serve cold.

Nutrition information per serving: Kcal: 72, Protein: 8.4g, Carbs: 21.2g, Fats: 1.4g

38.   Strawberry Lime Juice

Ingredients:

1 cup of strawberries, chopped

1 whole lime, peeled

1 small Granny Smith's apple, cored

1 whole lemon, peeled

2 oz coconut water

¼ tsp cinnamon, ground

Preparation:

Wash the strawberries and remove the stems. Cut into bite-sized pieces and fill the measuring cup. Reserve the rest for later.

Peel the lime and lemon. Cut each fruit in half and set aside.

Wash the apple and cut lengthwise in half. Remove the core and cut into small pieces. Set aside.

Now, combine strawberries, lime, lemon, and apple in a juicer and process until juiced. Transfer to a serving glass and stir in the coconut water and cinnamon.

Add some crushed ice and serve immediately.

Nutrition information per serving: Kcal: 122, Protein: 2.4g, Carbs: 39.7g, Fats: 0.9g

39.   Pineapple Orange Juice

Ingredients:

1 cup of pineapple, chunked

1 large orange, peeled

½ cup of spinach, torn

3 Brussels sprouts, halved

Preparation:

Using a sharp paring knife, cut the top of the pineapple. Gently remove all hard skin and slice it into thin slices. Fill the measuring cup and reserve the rest for later.

Peel the orange and divide into wedges. Cut each wedge in half and set aside.

Wash the spinach thoroughly under cold running water and torn with hands. Set aside.

Wash the Brussels sprouts and trim off the wilted leaves. Cut each in half and set aside.

Now, combine pineapple, orange, spinach, and Brussels sprouts in a juicer and process until well juiced. Transfer to a serving glass and refrigerate for 15 minutes before serving.

Enjoy!

Nutrition information per serving: Kcal: 172, Protein: 7.9g, Carbs: 52.7g, Fats: 1.1g

40.   Carrot Celery Juice

Ingredients:

1 large carrot, sliced

1 cup of celery, chopped

1 whole lemon, peeled

1 small Golden Delicious apple, cored

¼ tsp turmeric, ground

¼ tsp ginger, ground

Preparation:

Wash and peel the carrot. Cut into small slices and set aside.

Wash the celery and cut into small pieces. Set aside.

Peel the lemon and cut lengthwise in half. Set aside.

Wash the apple and cut in half. Remove the core and cut into bite-sized pieces. Set aside.

Now, combine carrot, celery, lemon, and apple in a juicer and process until juiced. Transfer to a serving glass and stir in the water, turmeric, and ginger. If you like, add some crushed ice.

Serve immediately.

Nutrition information per serving: Kcal: 105, Protein: 2.4g, Carbs: 32.8g, Fats: 0.7g

41.   Pear Cabbage Juice

Ingredients:

1 large pear, chopped

1 cup of purple cabbage, chopped

1 whole lemon, peeled

1 whole cucumber, sliced

Preparation:

Wash the pear and cut lengthwise in half. Remove the core and chop into small pieces. Set aside.

Wash the cabbage thoroughly under cold running water. Drain and chop into small pieces. Set aside.

Peel the lemon and cut lengthwise in half. Set aside.

Wash the cucumber and cut into thin slices. Set aside.

Now, combine pear, cabbage, lemon, and cucumber in a juicer. Process until well juiced. Transfer to a serving glass and serve immediately.

Enjoy!

Nutrition information per serving: Kcal: 173, Protein: 4.7g, Carbs: 57.9g, Fats: 0.9g

42. Cauliflower Tomato Juice

Ingredients:

1 cup of cauliflower, chopped

1 medium-sized tomato, chopped

½ cup of spring onions, chopped

½ cup of basil, torn

1 cup of cucumber, sliced

1 oz of water

Preparation:

Trim off the outer leaves of the cauliflower. Wash it and cut into small pieces. Fill the measuring cup and reserve the rest for later. Set aside.

Wash the tomato and place in a small bowl. Chop into small pieces and reserve the tomato juice while cutting. Set aside.

Wash the spring onions and basil. Chop into small pieces. Set aside.

Wash the cucumber and cut into thin slices. Fill the measuring cup and reserve the rest for later. Set aside.

Now, combine cauliflower, tomato, spring onions, basil, and cucumber in a juicer and process until well juiced. Transfer to a serving glass and stir in the water.

Serve cold.

Nutrition information per serving: Kcal: 51, Protein: 4.4g, Carbs: 13.9g, Fats: 0.7g

43.   Cantaloupe Strawberry Juice

Ingredients:

1 cup of cantaloupe, chopped

1 cup of strawberries, chopped

1 cup of banana, chunked

2 whole plums, chopped

¼ tsp of cinnamon, ground

Preparation:

Cut the cantaloupe in half. Scrape out the seeds and cut one one large wedge. Peel and chop into small pieces and fill the measuring cup. Wrap the rest in a plastic foil and refrigerate for later.

Wash the strawberries and remove the stems. Cut into bite-sized pieces and set aside.

Peel the banana and cut into chunks. Fill the measuring cup and reserve the rest. Set aside.

Wash the plums and cut each in half. Remove the pits and cut into small pieces. Set aside.

Now, combine cantaloupe, strawberries, banana, and plums in a juicer and process until juiced. Transfer to a serving glass and stir in the cinnamon.

Add some crushed ice and serve immediately.

Nutrition information per serving: Kcal: 249, Protein: 4.8g, Carbs: 73.1g, Fats: 1.5g

44. Swiss Chard Kale Juice

Ingredients:

2 cups of Swiss chard, torn

1 cup of fresh kale, torn

1 cup of pomegranate seeds

1 large orange, peeled

1 small Granny Smith's apple, cored

Preparation:

Combine Swiss chard and kale in a large colander. Rinse under cold running water and drain. Torn into small pieces and set aside.

Cut the top of the pomegranate fruit using a sharp paring knife. Slice down to each of the white membranes inside of the fruit. Pop the seeds into a measuring cup and set aside.

Peel the orange and divide into wedges. Cut each wedge in half and set aside.

Wash the apple and cut lengthwise in half. Remove the core and cut into bite-sized pieces. Set aside.

Now, combine Swiss chard, kale, pomegranate seeds, orange, and apple in a juicer and process until juiced. Transfer to a serving glass and add few ice cubes.

Serve immediately.

Nutrition information per serving: Kcal: 227, Protein: 7.9g, Carbs: 66.1g, Fats: 2.3g

45.   Pineapple Mango Juice

Ingredients:

1 cup of pineapple, chunked

1 cup of mango, chopped

1 cup of kale, torn

1 large orange, peeled

1 small ginger knob, chopped

Preparation:

Using a sharp paring knife, cut the top of the pineapple. Gently remove all hard skin and cut it into small chunks. Fill the measuring cup and reserve the rest for later.

Peel the mango and chop into small pieces. Fill the measuring cup and reserve the rest for later. Set aside.

Wash the kale thoroughly under cold running water. Drain and torn into small pieces. Set aside.

Peel the orange and divide into wedges. Cut each wedge in half and set aside.

Peel the ginger knob and cut into small pieces. Set aside.

Now, combine pineapple, mango, kale, orange, and ginger in a juicer and process until juiced. Transfer to a serving glass and refrigerate for 15 minutes before serving.

Enjoy!

Nutrition information per serving: Kcal: 258, Protein: 6.9g, Carbs: 74.9g, Fats: 1.7g

46.   Pepper Cabbage Juice

Ingredients:

1 large red bell pepper, chopped

1 cup of purple cabbage, chopped

1 cup of beets, sliced

1 cup of fresh spinach, torn

3 cherry tomatoes, halved

¼ tsp of salt

Preparation:

Wash the bell pepper and cut lengthwise in half. Remove the stem and seeds. Cut into small pieces and set aside.

Combine cabbage and spinach in a large colander. Rinse thoroughly under cold running water and drain. Torn into small pieces and set aside.

Wash the beets and trim off the green parts. Peel and cut into thin slices and fill the measuring cup. Reserve the rest for later.

Wash the cherry tomatoes and remove the stems. Cut into halves and set aside.

Now, combine bell pepper, cabbage, beets, spinach, and tomatoes in a juicer and process until juiced. Transfer to a serving glass and stir in the salt.

Serve immediately.

Nutrition information per serving: Kcal: 134, Protein: 11.5g, Carbs: 39.1g, Fats: 1.8g

47.   Blueberry Cucumber Juice

Ingredients:

1 cup of blueberries

1 cup of cucumber, sliced

1 cup of strawberries, chopped

1 cup of fresh mint, torn

1 large carrot, sliced

¼ tsp of cinnamon, ground

Preparation:

Wash the blueberries using a small colander. Drain and set aside.

Wash the cucumber and cut into thin slices. Fill the measuring cup and reserve the rest in the refrigerator.

Wash the strawberries and remove the stems. Chop into small pieces and set aside.

Wash the mint thoroughly under cold running water. Drain and torn into small pieces. Set aside.

Wash and peel the carrot. Cut into thin slices and set aside.

Now, combine blueberries, cucumber, strawberries, mint, and carrot in a juicer. Process until well juiced.

Transfer to a serving glass and stir in the cinnamon. Add some crushed ice and serve immediately!

Nutrition information per serving: Kcal: 141, Protein: 4g, Carbs: 45g, Fats: 1.3g

48.   Grape Cherry Juice

Ingredients:

2 cups of green grapes

1 cup of frozen cherries, thawed

1 small banana, peeled

1 whole lime, peeled

1 tbsp of coconut water

Preparation:

Rinse the grapes under cold running water and remove the stems. Set aside.

Peel the banana and cut into chunks. Set aside.

Peel the lime and cut lengthwise in half. Set aside

Now, combine grapes, cherries, banana, and lime in a juicer and process until juiced. Transfer to a serving glass and stir in the coconut water.

Serve immediately.

Nutrition information per serving: Kcal: 292, Protein: 4.1g, Carbs: 82.9g, Fats: 1.3g

49.   Lemon Leek Juice

Ingredients:

1 whole lemon, peeled

1 whole leek, chopped

1 whole lime, peeled

1 large orange, peeled

1 small green apple, cored

Preparation:

Peel the lemon and lime. Cut each fruit lengthwise in half and set aside.

Wash the leek and chop into small pieces. Set aside.

Peel the orange and divide into wedges. Cut each wedge in half and set aside.

Wash the apple and cut in half. Remove the core and cut into small pieces. Set aside.

Now, combine lemon, leek, lime, orange, and apple in a juicer and process until juiced. Transfer to a serving glass and refrigerate for 15 minutes before serving.

Enjoy!

Nutrition information per serving: Kcal: 205, Protein: 4.5g, Carbs: 62.9g, Fats: 0.9g

50.   Avocado Radish Juice

Ingredients:

1 cup of avocado, cubed

3 large radishes, chopped

1 small zucchini, sliced

1 cup of celery, chopped

1 cup of cucumber, sliced

¼ tsp of salt

1 oz of water

Preparation:

Peel the avocado and cut in half. Remove the pit and cut into small cubes. Fill the measuring cup and reserve the rest for later.

Wash the radishes and cut into small pieces. Set aside.

Wash the zucchini and cut into thin slices. Set aside.

Wash the celery and chop it into bite-sized pieces. Set aside.

Wash the cucumber and cut into thin slices. Fill the measuring cup and reserve the rest for later. Set aside.

Now, combine avocado, radishes, zucchini, celery, and cucumber in a juicer and process until juiced. Transfer to a serving glass and stir in the salt and water.

Serve cold.

Nutrition information per serving: Kcal: 235, Protein: 5.6g, Carbs: 22.3g, Fats: 22.6g

51.   Mango Kiwi Juice

Ingredients:

1 cup of mango, chopped

1 whole kiwi, peeled

1 small Grany Smith's apple, cored

1 small ginger knob, peeled

2 oz of coconut water

Preparation:

Peel the mango and cut into small pieces. Fill the measuring cup and reserve the rest for later.

Peel the kiwi and cut lengthwise in half. Set aside.

Wash the apple and cut lengthwise in half. Remove the core and cut into small pieces. Set aside.

Peel the ginger knob and cut into small pieces. Set aside.

Now, combine mango, kiwi, apple, and ginger in a juicer and process until juiced. Transfer to a serving glass and stir in the coconut water. Add some crushed ice and serve immediately.

Enjoy!

Nutrition information per serving: Kcal: 196, Protein: 2.8g, Carbs: 55.5g, Fats: 1.3g

52. Broccoli Pumpkin Juice

Ingredients:

1 cup of broccoli, chopped

1 cup of pumpkin, cubed

1 whole lemon, peeled

1 cup of fennel, chopped

1 cup of cucumber, sliced

Preparation:

Wash the broccoli and trim off the outer leaves. Cut into bite-sized pieces and fill the measuring cup. Reserve the rest for later.

Cut the top of a pumpkin. Cut lengthwise in half and then scrape out the seeds. Cut one large wedge and peel it. Cut into small cubes and fill the measuring cup. Reserve the rest in the refrigerator.

Peel the lemon and cut lengthwise in half. Set aside.

Trim off the outer wilted layers of the fennel. Roughly chop it and fill the measuring cup. Reserve the rest for later.

Wash the cucumber and cut into thin slices. Fill the measuring cup and reserve the rest in the refrigerator. Set aside.

Now, combine broccoli, pumpkin, lemon, fennel, and cucumber in a juicer and process until well juiced. Transfer to a serving glass and add some crushed ice.

Serve immediately.

Nutrition information per serving: Kcal: 196, Protein: 2.8g, Carbs: 55.5g, Fats: 1.3g

ADDITIONAL TITLES FROM THIS AUTHOR

70 Effective Meal Recipes to Prevent and Solve Being Overweight: Burn Fat Fast by Using Proper Dieting and Smart Nutrition

By

Joe Correa CSN

48 Acne Solving Meal Recipes: The Fast and Natural Path to Fixing Your Acne Problems in Less Than 10 Days!

By

Joe Correa CSN

41 Alzheimer's Preventing Meal Recipes: Reduce or Eliminate Your Alzheimer's Condition in 30 Days or Less!

By

Joe Correa CSN

70 Effective Breast Cancer Meal Recipes: Prevent and Fight Breast Cancer with Smart Nutrition and Powerful Foods

By

Joe Correa CSN

www.ingramcontent.com/pod-product-compliance
Lightning Source LLC
Chambersburg PA
CBHW030257030426
42336CB00009B/417